For my partner,

best friend,

and wife – Lori

REFLECTIONS
on the hands of a nurse

A book of prayers and reflections for nurses
By Mark Darby, RN

Published by Surprise Publishing
2917 North 49th Street • Omaha NE 68104

Cover Design, Layout and Poster Design by Carol Sayers
and the great folks at Diversity Print and Graphics LLC
Omaha NE • www.diversityprint.com

Cataloging Information

Darby, Mark
Reflections on the Hands of a Nurse:
a book of poems and prayers for nurses
by Mark Darby First Edition
160 pages
ISBN 1890523-06-2

Library of Congress Control Number: 2004095902

Introduction

This project started several years ago when I was frustrated at work. Rather than my normal griping and complaining, I said a quick prayer. It seemed as if Somebody was listening because the shift went better than I expected. Since then, I have spent some time exploring the spirituality of Nursing. It seems that nurses, many subconsciously, use their spirituality to survive and thrive in today's world of healthcare. This book is the result of conversations I have had with nurses about their beliefs, their prayers, and their hopes for Nursing.

Section 1 is a collection of prayers concerning common situations in a nurse's career. Section 2 is about the power of "story" and how to discover your own story. Section 3 contains a variety of reflections that were written about Nursing and several Nursing specialties.

Each of these sections is independent of the other. This book does not have to be read in any particular order. Some have told me that they have read one prayer a day and used the questions before each as a part of their daily prayer. Others have used Section 2 during all day programs and retreats.

All these ways are valid, so long as they satisfy you, the reader.

Mark Darby, RN
Omaha, NE

Table of Contents

Table of Contents (Continued)

prayers
chapter one

Prayer for an Obnoxious Co-Worker

"Life was going along fine until she started in griping and complaining. Nothing was right. I was hoping that she would just shut up and go away. But, she stayed right where she was, continuing to gripe."

From a 3-11
Medical Surgical Nurse

Did you ever experience a time when another co-worker was truly acting obnoxious? It may have seemed as if you were breathing fresh air that suddenly became polluted by output from an old industrial plant. How did you cope in this situation?

Being sensitive to someone else's emotional state can help us be good nurses. However, when dealing with an obnoxious co-worker, we must limit our sensitivity. Handling this person objectively allows you to decide how to react to his (her) negative emotions.

Questions for Reflection

1. Describe a time when you worked with an obnoxious co-worker.

   _____

   _____

   _____

   _____

   _____

2. How did you handle this situation?

   _____

   _____

   _____

   _____

   _____

3. What would you like to do in the future?

   _____

   _____

   _____

   _____

   _____

Prayer for an Obnoxious Co-Worker

*Life was going along fine until he (she)
    started in on it.*

*I keep hoping he (she) will just go away,
    but I know that's not the answer.
I still have to work with him (her).*

*Forgiving God, I pray that the situation will change.
I want to be better able to cope.
I pray that
    I will not be affected by the waves of
        negativity, and that
    I will be able to confront him (her)
        when I need to.*

*I honestly hope and pray for his (her) health and
well-being, and that You will bless his (her) life.*

Prayer for
When I Am Obnoxious

Every once in awhile, you wake up thinking that you deserve a day to gripe and complain. It just seems that things have not been going your way lately so you deserve to be in a bad mood. At first, it feels good. You can finally tell those other drivers exactly what you're thinking. You can put on a "Don't mess with me, Buddy" look. Sometimes those days seem to be the very thing you need.

But, there is a downside to griping and complaining. Griping rarely helps us feel better in the long run. When we complain, we can end up hurting someone else and having to apologize the next day. In addition, sometimes we gripe and complain to avoid making necessary changes in our lives. It is easier to complain than to change.

Questions for Reflection

1. Describe a day when you were crabby.

   _____

   _____

   _____

   _____

   _____

2. What happened to contribute to these feelings?

   _____

   _____

   _____

   _____

   _____

3. After you moaned and groaned awhile,
   did things improve?

   _____

   _____

   _____

   _____

   _____

Prayer for When
I Am Obnoxious

I thought I deserved just one day.
I wanted to get it out of my system.
Then I realized I couldn't get it out.
   It wouldn't leave.
The more I griped, the worse I felt.

I pray that this will stop.
I don't want to feel like this anymore.
I want to feel more like me.

I pray that You will help me find a better,
   more effective way
   to make the changes I need.

I also pray for all those people who were the
   victims of my griping.
I pray that they will be healed,
and that they will forgive me.

Prayer for an Obnoxious Physician

There are a lot of movies and TV shows made about doctors and nurses. In them, you will see the dedicated physician buoyed by the brilliant, but submissive nurse. These images distort reality.

The bottom line is that both physicians and nurses have complex jobs that attract a wide range of personalities. Sometimes we may have a bad interaction with an individual. When that happens, we need to be careful not to generalize. We must not lump all physicians into one broad category.

But, there are those MDs that seem to go out of their way to be obnoxious. Encountering these MDs can create paralyzing feelings. Prayer can help to release you from this paralysis.

Questions for Reflection

1. Describe a time when you had a difficult
    experience with a physician.

    _____

    _____

    _____

    _____

    _____

2. How did you cope with that MD? Did it affect
    your relationship with other physicians?

    _____

    _____

    _____

    _____

3. How would you prefer to relate to difficult
    physicians?

    _____

    _____

    _____

    _____

Prayer for an Obnoxious Physician

I'm so mad right now!
That doctor was condescending and patronizing.
His (her) tone of voice was unnecessary.
I am fuming about not saying what I wanted to say.

I pray that this hot anger will leave me.
I want to be free from the control
    the anger holds over me.
I pray this relationship will change and
    that I will not be the subject of this tirade again.

I pray that change will occur
not only in myself,
but also in the physician, so that this
    will not happen again.

Prayer for When You're Tired and on the Late Shift

This work can wear on your soul. Sometimes when you look at the clock, you can't believe how slowly the hours are passing. It is times like these when the work is most difficult. You must still perform at the same level, but your abilities are compromised. How do you make an assessment when all you want to do is go to sleep?

The late shift has many advantages such as no bosses, an intimate staff, and a relaxed atmosphere. But there are times when you are fighting your body's natural rhythms and you ask, "Why do I work this shift?"

There is always the hope of a second wind when tiredness seems to float away.   Many things can bring it about: a quick break, a cup of hot chocolate, accomplishing a task, or a quick prayer. Thankfully, before you know it, your shift ends and you suddenly find your way home.

Questions for Reflection

1. Remind yourself of three good reasons you work these odd hours.

   _____

   _____

   _____

   _____

   _____

2. What have you accomplished this shift that made you glad to be working these hours?

   _____

   _____

   _____

   _____

   _____

3. What are two things you will do when you get home to ensure you get your proper rest?

   _____

   _____

   _____

   _____

   _____

Prayer for When You're Tired and on the Late Shift

I just looked at the clock right now
    and I can't believe how little time has passed.
I am exhausted.

I shuffle from patient to patient.
I just want to sleep, and
I can't stand the taste of coffee.

Lord, help me make it through this shift.

I pray that my lack of energy will not cause
    a mistake to occur.
Help me to not be obsessed with the clock.
Give me enough energy, judgment, and alertness
    to provide good care.

And when I finally go home, give me a
    good night's (day's) rest.

Prayer for When You're Burnt Out

We all reach a point when we just want to quit. At the end of a very stressful day, we say, "I am never coming back." Most of the time, these feelings are transitory and we return the next day. At other times, the bad days won't go away. They hang around our neck like a heavy yoke that drags us down to the ground.

As a protective mechanism, when the days become especially onerous, we start to devalue the work we do, the people we serve, and, eventually, ourselves. We fail to recognize the reasons we were first attracted to Nursing, and the people we serve become less than human.

At this stage, three things can happen. First, people usually leave an organization. Second, and possibly worse, people stay with an organization they should have left. Or, third, people choose to remember what excited them about Nursing in the first place, recalling the special privilege it is to care for our patients.

Questions for Reflection

1. What is the most important thing you do at work?

    _____

    _____

    _____

    _____

    _____

2. What have you done to take care of yourself
    today? What would you like to do?

    _____

    _____

    _____

    _____

    _____

3. How long have you had these burnt out
    feelings? What are some of the main causes of
    your burnout?

    _____

    _____

    _____

    _____

    _____

Prayer for
When You're Burnt Out

I just don't want to work today.
I don't want to be here
or be doing what I am doing.
I would prefer to sell shoes door-to-door.

When I come to work, it seems to eat a hole
*   in my soul.*

However,
*   when I remember why I became a nurse, I want*
*   to give quality care and make a difference.*

So, Nurturing God,
*   I pray for healing to make my soul whole.*
*   I pray for a return of energy and enjoyment.*

Help me to resolve the factors that have made
*   the burnout worse.*
Help me to go on feeling energized and make
*   my efforts worthwhile.*

Prayer for Accepting My Limitations

There are times when we realize that we cannot do any more, and yet, we desperately wish that we could do something else. We may think that one more intervention or one alteration in a personality would make everything okay, but this type of thinking leads nowhere.

Worry has never changed anything. Obsession. Regret. Shame. None of these ever altered the present. When the reality is that we cannot do anything else, the only option is acceptance.

Accepting our limitations means we understand we are not superhuman. When we have done all that a human being can reasonably be expected to do, we have reached our limits. Nurses can forget this plain, simple fact. We are humans doing a demanding job. There will always be patients for whom we wish more could be done. Whether it is a dialysis patient in the clinic or an oncology patient in the home, the health of some patients is beyond our control.

Acceptance does not mean that we fail to strive for excellence at patient care. Nurses have, and should have, high standards of care. We should do all we can to look after the people in our care. It is precisely for this reason that we need to accept our limits. Acceptance will redirect our efforts and energies towards what we can do, rather than focusing on what we wish we could do.

Questions for Reflection

1. Recall a time you wished you could do more for
    a patient but could not. Describe it here.

    _____
    _____
    _____
    _____
    _____

2. Accepting your limits is different than poor
    performance. What do you think some of the
    differences are?

    _____
    _____
    _____
    _____
    _____

3. What do you do when you have reached your
    limits?

    _____
    _____
    _____
    _____
    _____

Prayer for Accepting My Limitations

One thing I know for sure is that
  there will always be more:
more need than I can fulfill,
more than I can ever do.

Yet, I don't feel like I can stop.

I think if I just spend a little more time,
I could satisfy the need and
fulfill all the demands.
It hurts me to think that I can't do it all.

Sometimes I stay so focused
on all I want to do that
I stop doing what I can do.

Comforting God,
  help me to know my limits,
  to do what I can do well,
  and to be at peace
  with what I cannot do.

Prayer about Challenges

Being good at what you do is important. Nurses are motivated when they have the opportunity to learn new things, to take on difficult tasks, and to improve upon what we know how to do. Nurses like being challenged. However, a challenge should not be confused with endurance.

Working a long, hard shift can be called a challenge, but it's more likely to be an act of endurance. We should never be satisfied with just enduring through work. Healthcare is too rich with learning opportunities to settle for simply being alive at the end of a shift.

There are always days that are long and hard. But, there are also numerous opportunities in each day to gain experience that will make you a better person.

Questions for Reflection

1. What makes one experience a challenge and another simply something to be endured?

   _____

   _____

   _____

   _____

   _____

2. When was your last challenge?

   _____

   _____

   _____

   _____

3. In the future, what is one thing about Nursing you would like to learn more about?

   _____

   _____

   _____

   _____

   _____

Prayer about Challenges

I like being able to do something
that no one else can do.
I like doing difficult things well.
I love operating on intuition.

And so,
I thank You, God of Knowledge, for giving me
a job that allows me the opportunity
to do such things.

I pray that I will continue to look for new
opportunities to become better at what I do.

Prayer for When You're Angry at the System

There are situations where everyone agrees that a particular course of action should be taken, yet nothing is done. When you ask, "Why?" everyone blames someone else. All you hear is excuses. Someone will say, "That's just the way it is."

When this happens and you get angry, to whom do you direct your anger? How do you put a face on the bureaucracy? How do you find the person who can change the decision and make an exception? While such change is possible, it oftentimes requires patience and planning.

Meanwhile, you must still care for patients as best you can. Anger at some faceless crowd can hamper good care. However, anger can also help you make long-term changes in the healthcare system.

Questions for Reflection

1. When was the last time you felt angry at some part of the healthcare bureaucracy?

    _____

    _____

    _____

    _____

    _____

2. What did you do to deal with those feelings?

    _____

    _____

    _____

    _____

    _____

3. How would you like to handle those feelings next time?

    _____

    _____

    _____

    _____

    _____

Prayer for When You are Angry at the System

Somewhere
Someone made a decision
that affected my patient.

It's frustrating when you try to do
something and all you hear is,

"The insurance company won't cover it",
  "There is not enough money",
"It is not necessary", or
  "We just don't do that."

How do you fight against someone you cannot see?

Yet, I know and believe
there is a greater Power
in control of all things,
and that Power creates justice.

God of Justice, I pray for my patient and
  for me as we do the best we can.
Create a safe place for us.
Ensure that I can give the best care possible.

Prayer for Someone Undergoing Chemotherapy

Chemotherapy has such a neat sounding name: very modern and efficient. But, chemotherapy can be messy. It is more than taking a medication for a few hours and then going home. Chemotherapy involves everything from hope to nausea.

Each person's chemotherapy experience is unique. It is something you cannot understand completely unless you have been through it. As nurses, we must try to be sympathetic to the ways that patients handle their treatment. If we get so busy that they are treated like cattle, we will be unable to care for our patients as individuals.

Our busyness can occur for many reasons, ranging from the number of treatments to the demands of the physicians. It can also be used as a protective mechanism. Regardless of the reason, it is important to remember that chemotherapy is more than the medication a patient receives. It affects their entire life.

Questions for Reflection

1. What are some of the challenges faced by all chemotherapy patients?

   _____

   _____

   _____

   _____

   _____

2. Recall a patient you know who has undergone chemotherapy. What are some of the unique needs he or she had?

   _____

   _____

   _____

   _____

   _____

3. What are some ways you can increase the support you give to the patients undergoing chemotherapy?

   _____

   _____

   _____

   _____

Prayer for Someone Undergoing Chemotherapy

We (I) pray today for _____, who is about to undergo chemotherapy.

*We (I) pray that the medication will be effective, and that the side effects,
especially _____,
will be minimal.*

*We (I) know that You, God of Health,
are more powerful than cancer.
We pray that You will make
Your power known by causing this treatment
to be successful.*

*We also ask that You support the family
and friends of _____.*

Give strength and encouragement where it is needed.

*As they help care for _____,
let them know that
You can be of aid and comfort to them
and will help meet their needs too.*

Prayer for the Beginning of a Day at a Clinic

Today dozens, perhaps hundreds, of people will come through the door. Everyone will have their own problems and their own experiences. Everyone will want answers to their questions.

You will see them all, and every one of them could potentially become a blur. When you hear the same question over and over again, it may become hard to treat people as individuals.

Rather than letting it become a blur, the day could be unique. It could give you something to laugh at. It could hold something meaningful. It could be a day when you impact someone in a special way. It is easier to be open to the unique aspects of the day if we spend a few quiet minutes before the start of the day.

Questions for Reflection

1. When you go to your doctor's office, how would you like to be treated?

   _____
   _____
   _____
   _____
   _____

2. What is the most frequent complaint you will likely see today?

   _____
   _____
   _____
   _____
   _____

3. What will you do to address the unique needs of your patients?

   _____
   _____
   _____
   _____
   _____

Prayer for the Beginning of a Day at a Clinic

I pray that all my patients will be able
  to receive the best care
I have to offer.

Help me to not be too distracted
or too busy to treat all people
with concern.

I pray specifically for the one
who will try my patience
and make it difficult for me.

Help me to be calm and courteous.

Gracious God, help me make a difference today.

Prayer for a Patient Who Experiences Bad Side Effects

"Side effects are to be expected. Certain side effects have to be tolerated when you take a medication." How many times have you said something like this to a patient?

Side effects can mean something totally different to a patient than they do to a health care professional. I once told a patient that the only side effect that she may experience would be a "little diarrhea". The next day, after having to spend several hours on the toilet, she wanted me to define in exact terms what "little" really meant.

While this was taken in good humor, she did have a point. When you don't personally have to experience the side effects, it is easy to discount the impact they can have on people's lives.

Some medications have tremendous side effects, but they may also be the only option left to save a life.

There are times when we have to make difficult decisions. I wonder what decision I would make if I had to choose between a terminal illness becoming worse or throwing up all day?

As patients make a decision about how to deal with side effects, they need the support and knowledge of nurses. We have to be prepared to listen to and try to understand the patient.

Questions for Reflection

1. What is the best way to tell a patient about possible side effects?

   _____

   _____

   _____

   _____

   _____

2. How can you encourage a patient to ask questions?

   _____

   _____

   _____

   _____

   _____

3. How do you react when a patient decides to quit taking a medication because of a side effect?

   _____

   _____

   _____

   _____

   _____

Prayer for a Patient Who Experiences Bad Side Effects

A medication we gave
  was supposed to help,
  but has caused this patient
  to be in discomfort.

I pray this will either stop or become tolerable.

May he (she) experience relief.
Help us to know if there is any other way
  we can help this patient
  and to do what we can do to assist him (her).

I also ask that as the treatment progresses,
the patient will experience health and healing.

Prayer for When You're Told to Do Something That Just Doesn't Make Sense

One day I came to work and read a memo. "Important!" it said.

"The policy regarding the documentation of the Environmental Assessment form, implemented last week, has been changed and updated. Please disregard the previous procedure regarding the Environmental Assessment form and start using the attached form immediately." The information was already collected on two other forms. This change, the third one in six months, doubled the time it took to complete the form.

In healthcare, we have to separate the silly from the essential. When giving care, we need to focus on what is essential. There are other times to deal with the stuff that doesn't make sense.

Questions for Reflection

1. How do you react when you read a memo that does not make sense?

   _____

   _____

   _____

   _____

   _____

2. How do you address such issues professionally?

   _____

   _____

   _____

   _____

   _____

3. What is your favorite story of having to do something impractical?

   _____

   _____

   _____

   _____

   _____

Prayer for When You're Told to Do Something That Just Doesn't Make Sense

I pray that I will give good care today despite this stuff that makes me mad.

I pray that You, God of Patience, will help me deal with the negative feelings that come along with it.

Help me to deal with this at an appropriate time and place.
Help me to remember and be guided by my own competence.

I also pray for whomever thought this up.
Give them insight into the effect this has on my job.

Prayer for Someone Who Does Not Breathe Well

Breathing. In and out. In and out. Hundreds of times an hour. Most people go through their day assuming their lungs will work. We nurses don't.

We know what can go wrong. We have learned to deal with the problems associated with not breathing well. In fact, we have dealt with it so often that you could say we have "mechanized" breathing. When the diaphragm will not work, we use a ventilator. When there is a blockage, we will make a new opening.

The mechanization of breathing can give us a sense of control. We can come to believe that technology can be the solution to all problems. But technology has its limits.

What do we do about the helplessness felt by a person whose lungs don't work? What do we do with the panic of a parent whose child is turning blue? Where are the machines for these feelings?

There are no machines. There is only our caring, our empathy, and our ability to give support. Remember, we deal with more than lungs. We must deal with the mind and spirits of whole, living people who do not breathe well.

Questions for Reflection

1. Think about the last time you looked past the mechanics of breathing to the wonder of the human body. What impressed you?

   _____

   _____

   _____

   _____

   _____

2. How are you able to give comfort to those who do not breathe well?

   _____

   _____

   _____

   _____

   _____

3. Do you take your own breathing for granted?

   _____

   _____

   _____

   _____

   _____

Prayer for Someone
Who Does Not Breathe Well

Breathing always seems so easy
  until you can't do it.

Retractions, wheezing, and gasps are all
  reminders that some people are thankful
  for each breath they take.

And now, as I care for someone
  who struggles for each breath,
I pray You will open their
  bronchi and alveoli and
  fill them with Your blessing.

Ease their struggle as much as You can.
Make each effort successful.
Give oxygen where it is most needed
  and remove the toxins that accumulate.

Help me, Lord, to remember my own breathing
  with a grateful heart.

Prayer for a Rehab Patient

Medicine is obsessed with progress. There is nothing better than a rapidly escalating improvement line. However, our patients don't listen to trend lines.

Minimal, but steady, progress describes some patients. Long plateaus with bursts of accomplishment describe others. The only factor that does not change for either type of progress is the need for care. We have to provide care steadily and professionally, no matter how steep or how flat the trend line is for the patient.

When faced with multiple tasks, we often look for ways to take short cuts. "What is it that we can get by with not doing today?" we may ask. When dealing with our patients, we have to answer, "Nothing." With patients who make slower progress, we may think that one little treatment can be skipped. However, we must be thorough in what we do so that, in time, patients can make the progress they are capable of making.

Questions for Reflection

1. Think of the last time a rehab patient you cared for made some progress or was able to maintain some functioning. Describe it here.

   _____

   _____

   _____

   _____

   _____

2. How can we increase our awareness of the slow, steady progress made by some of our patients?

   _____

   _____

   _____

   _____

3. Is there anything in your life that makes slow, steady progress?

   _____

   _____

   _____

   _____

Prayer for a Rehab Patient

Just a little more movement,
  a little more independence,
That is what I hope for him(her).

Just a little more.
  He (She) is trying as hard as he (she) can,
  making a little progress each day.

I hope and pray that You will
Give him (her) strength
  and increase his (her) tolerance of pain,

Protect him (her) from too much
  discouragement and hopelessness,
and over time, I pray he(she) will be the
  best he(she) is able to be.

Prayer of Thanksgiving for Making a Difference

We talk about the five rights: right patient, right route, right medicine, right time, and right dose. These five rights protect patients by avoiding medication errors. However, there are another five rights that are equally important. They are being the right person, at the right time, with the right knowledge, given to the right patient, in the right way.

When this happens, we have the skills necessary to give the people we serve exactly what they need. We relieve pain, give knowledge, empower, and enhance health and functioning. We have made a difference. When these times occur, they are the best experiences in Nursing.

Unfortunately, these days and these treasures can quickly be forgotten. They can be lost in the hullabaloo that is healthcare, unless we take time to remember.

Questions for Reflection

1. Remember a time when you made a difference. Describe it here.

   _____

   _____

   _____

   _____

   _____

2. How often do you have these experiences in a given week?

   _____

   _____

   _____

   _____

   _____

3. Here is an optional assignment: The next time you work, tell yourself to be mindful of times when you make a difference. At the end of the day, reflect on those experiences.

   _____

   _____

   _____

   _____

   _____

Prayer of Thanksgiving
for Making a Difference

Today I made a difference.
I was the right person,
   at the right time,
   with the right knowledge,
   given to the right patient,
   in the right way.

I want to take a moment to recall
   that experience right now.

I want to recapture that moment now
   so it won't be forgotten.

I want to remember and say, "Thank You, God."
   Thanks for letting me have that experience.

Help me to be open to the next opportunity.

Prayer for a Special Patient

We are taught about the value of having a professional demeanor and keeping an objective viewpoint, no matter who the patient may be. This shield can protect us from being drained emotionally.

Occasionally, this shield is penetrated. In the middle of a busy day, our curiosity gets piqued. We begin to notice a particular patient and we become involved. We take a greater interest in this case than in others, and we begin to hope that this person will be well.

Getting more involved can be risky for health professionals. We might be disappointed, but we can also find joy that can help us in hard times.

Questions for Reflection

1. Remember a special patient. Describe him here.

    _____

    _____

    _____

    _____

    _____

2. What type of patient impacts you?

    _____

    _____

    _____

    _____

    _____

3. When you allow a patient to become special, how
    does it help you be a better nurse?

    _____

    _____

    _____

    _____

    _____

Prayer for a Special Patient

I don't know why,
  but this patient is special.
He (she) broke through the professional distance.

He (she) made me cry and laugh,
  and I felt better.

I was taken care of today.
On some days I only give,
  but today I received, and I am glad for it.

Prayer for a Recovery from Surgery

When someone goes to the recovery room after surgery, they are neatly draped. They almost resemble a Christmas package. We have seen it so often that it has become routine, and we can easily forget the enormity of what happened to the person inside. A human being has just had their flesh cut open and tissue excised. In any other setting, this would be deadly. Yet, combined with skill and expertise, such actions can bring healing.

We need to remember that it is not our actions, but the blessings our actions bring that heal. Recovery has become somewhat like an assembly line where people come and go very quickly. However, we can still pause to take a brief moment and ask for further assistance with the work we do.

Questions for Reflection

1. What does a person most need to successfully recover from surgery?

   _____

   _____

   _____

   _____

   _____

2. When you think of the recovery process, what amazes you the most?

   _____

   _____

   _____

   _____

   _____

3. If you were a patient in recovery, how would you like to be cared for?

   _____

   _____

   _____

   _____

   _____

Prayer for a Recovery from Surgery

Now that my patient is all situated,
the IV lines are flowing,
the monitors are working,

and I have done what I can,
I ask that You, God of Healing, will be with him
*   (her) during the process of recovery.*

I ask for returning strength
and functioning.

During the time when
*   he (she) is most weak,*
*   lend him (her) Your strength and support.*

Bless the efforts of the medical team
*   and bless the family.*
Guide him (her)
*   in a return to full health.*

Prayer Before a Surgery

When I was in surgery once, I noticed a middle-aged woman who was about to go in for a cardiac operation. Her family had left her at the doorway. As she passed me on the gurney, she looked frightened, as if she had entered a whole new world.

When you encounter surgical venues on a daily basis, they become familiar. We get used to seeing people cut open and anesthetized. However, what is a regular occurrence for healthcare professionals can be a life-changing event for those not familiar with it.

Numerous studies show the positive effects of reassurance on surgical patients. We should remember that these patients will only get such reassurances from us.

Questions for Reflection

1. Have you or a family member ever been to surgery? How did it feel?

    _____

    _____

    _____

    _____

    _____

2. What are some of the aspects of surgery that can cause people to feel uneasy?

    _____

    _____

    _____

    _____

    _____

3. What do you do to provide comfort at these times?

    _____

    _____

    _____

    _____

    _____

Prayer Before a Surgery

We do a lot of these surgeries
  so they seem ordinary to me.
I want to take a moment to remember
  that this is extraordinary for this family.

As they wait for the end of this procedure,
I pray that You will be with them.

Give them what they need to handle
  the outcome of this surgery.

Make the wait not seem so long.
Lord, please give comfort to all those who need it

Prayer for an Understaffed Shift

Nothing can change your attitude more than working
a shift that is short-handed. On a particular evening
shift, two people had called in sick, leaving us
desperately short of talent. It was then that I began
to feel overwhelmed. I was responsible for the safety
of many more people than I had expected to be. I
was also scared that someone would get hurt and
there would be nothing I could do to stop it.

There are really two questions to think about when
you're in this situation. First, how do you get through
this shift? And second, could this have been prevented?
We often concentrate on only answering the first
question. We have to remember that the second
question also needs to be answered. If there is a
pattern within your organization of short staffing, it
must be dealt with in some way.

Luckily, I was working for a good organization, and
short staffing was not the usual pattern. So, we got
through that night by working hard and offering up
the prayer that follows.

Questions for Reflection

1. Recall the last time you worked short staffed. What happened?

   _____

   _____

   _____

   _____

   _____

2. How do you deal with short staffing?

   _____

   _____

   _____

   _____

3. Have you ever worked in a facility where short staffing was a pattern? What did you do about it?

   _____

   _____

   _____

   _____

Prayer for an Understaffed Shift

We're short of staff today,
and some of the folks who are here
don't want to be.

But, the demand is high,
requests are coming in,
and people are hurting.
Then there is also all that paperwork.
I'm scared I might hurt someone.

I ask that You, God of Strength and Energy,
be with me today.

Keep me focused on caring and assisting.

Make sure everyone is well and safe.
Give me the strength to deal
with the cause of this short staffing effectively.

And for now,
Lord, help me make it through this shift.

Prayer for Someone Who Has Died

Death is not something we like to spend time thinking about. As nurses, we can see a great many patients die. Often times, all this death just wears us down and leads to burnout. But, it's important to remember that death can also be a gift.

The dying patients I have worked with, especially those in hospice care, have taught me a great deal. Not to waste time. Not to be bothered by the little things. To make sure you say what you mean.

I guess, all things being equal, I would rather care for people who live. However, because I have looked after many who have died, I have thought more about my own death and what I want to accomplish before I leave this place. It has also caused me to think of how I would like to be cared for when I am dying, which has resulted in helping me give better care.

Questions for Reflection

1. Who was the last person you cared for that died? Describe that person here.

    _____

    _____

    _____

    _____

    _____

2. How did this person's death affect you?

    _____

    _____

    _____

    _____

    _____

3. What did you learn from that patient?

    _____

    _____

    _____

    _____

    _____

Prayer for Someone Who Has Died

*A few minutes ago, he (she) was alive and
    now he (she) is dead.
He (she) has gone to someplace we can
    only dream about.*

Despite our best efforts, he (she) didn't survive.

I ask You to ease their journey to a new place.

*Please give comfort to the family
    and friends who loved him (her),
    grew with him (her),
    and cared for him (her) while
    he (she) was ill.*

Prayer for a Person in Pain

Pain is so contradictory. In some people, the smallest amount of pain cripples. In others, a great deal of pain is gracefully endured. As nurses, we see pain uniquely. With our empathy, we are acutely aware of people in pain – almost as if we are experiencing the pain ourselves.

We try pills, shots, therapeutic touch, cold and warmth, repositioning, and many other ways to relieve pain. Perhaps we also need to ask assistance from God in our efforts to relieve pain.

All the efforts and tools we use to relieve pain would only be enhanced with help from God. When you ask God for assistance in pain relief, you may not get what you expected. One patient with crippling pain had tried all the treatments that were recommended with little relief. The side effects from some of the medications were intolerable.

Then one day, she seemed better. During the
assessment, I asked her about pain levels. She replied,
"It's a 7-8." Yet, she was outgoing, engaged and
enjoying life. She told me, she had grown frustrated
with the medications and, almost in desperation,
turned to God to ask for assistance. "The pain is still
there," she said. "I just seem to cope with it better
when I pray every day."

All the medications, all the technology, all our
powerful medical knowledge was ineffective. But the
age old method that didn't require a prescription
made a difference.

Questions for Reflection

1. Have you ever had a time when you felt frustrated because you could not relieve someone's pain? Describe it here.

   _____
   _____
   _____
   _____
   _____

2. Describe a person you encountered who coped with pain gracefully.

   _____
   _____
   _____
   _____
   _____

3. Recall a person you know who has chronic pain. What did he do to cope?

   _____
   _____
   _____
   _____
   _____

Prayer for a Person in Pain

Lord, _____ is in pain.

This discomfort is one of the most important
   experiences of his (her) life today.

We have tried many ways to relieve the pain.
We ask You now to do what You can to
   minimize this discomfort and to help
   _____ cope with the pain.

Pain is powerful, Lord. But help us
   to remember that You are stronger than pain,

And that You can give hope and comfort
   in all experiences, even pain.

Prayer for a Heart Patient

The heart holds a certain fascination for people.
Historically, it was thought to be the source of love
and fidelity. The heart is also the symbol of
Valentine's Day for millions of Hallmark card buyers.
But, nurses see it as something else.

Nurses know the heart differently than other people.
We don't think of the heart in a superficial way.
We have heard it with a stethoscope, felt a pulse with
our fingers, and maybe we have seen one during
surgery. These assessments create an intimacy with
the heart that few people know.

But with intimacy can come familiarity, and the
familiar can be taken for granted. The heart is a
source of life for human beings. Remembering this
helps us to retain awe for the human heart, for its
constant beating and pumping that others can take
for granted.

Questions for Reflection

1. Do you remember the first time you heard the human heart? What was your reaction?

_____

_____

_____

_____

_____

2. How did you react the first time you heard an abnormal heart rate?

_____

_____

_____

_____

_____

3. Think about the process it takes to restore a human heart that has stopped. How would a non-medical person describe this event?

_____

_____

_____

_____

_____

Prayer for a Heart Patient

Life-Giving God, You have created the heart
and it is a masterpiece.
Its fidelity to the task of pumping blood is
constant, until interrupted by an illness or injury.

I pray about such a heart now.
_____ has a damaged heart.

We can not assume that it will function
automatically today.

As we attempt to restore the heart and the person
to health, we ask that You will recreate the rate
and rhythm that is necessary for life.

Place Your hand on this chest and encourage the
heart to beat routinely again.

Help us to be grateful for Your handiwork
and to not take the beat for granted.

Prayer Before Inserting an IV

I remember a nurse named Eloise. She had the "magic touch." She had the ability to insert an IV needle into any arm - no matter what.

She seemed to be able to know the exact vein by sight, create confidence with her presence, and insert the needle just the right length without pain or infiltration.

I, on the other hand, could not insert an IV into a garden hose without breaking the needle.

When I asked Eloise how she did it with such skill, she replied, "I do two things. I practice a lot. And right before I start, I say a little prayer." This prayer is dedicated to Eloise.

Questions for Reflection

1. What do you do to improve your IV technique?

   _____

   _____

   _____

   _____

   _____

2. If you are really good at inserting an IV, how would you teach this skill to others?

   _____

   _____

   _____

   _____

   _____

3. If you are not very proficient at this skill, what would you like to know from an expert if you had the chance to ask?

   _____

   _____

   _____

   _____

   _____

Prayer Before Inserting an IV

I am about to insert an IV.

*Guide my hand. Help me to be sensitive
     enough to find the vein and to insert the needle
     just far enough.*

*Help the fluids delivered through this port
     bring health and healing.*

Prayer for an Alzheimer's Patient

Memory is a fleeting thing. Home. Parents. The way your name sounds. All are so deeply embedded in our brains that they form the foundation that defines who we are. Alzheimer's Disease can cause you to lose this foundation. Still, some memories remain strong to the very end.

Joan was 72, and had been suffering from Alzheimer's Disease for 10 years when I got to know her in the nursing home. Her husband, Henry, who was in poor health but not confused, also lived at the home. Joan would become very agitated when anyone would get too close to her.

However, one thing always calmed her down - the sight of her husband. Just looking at Henry soothed her and brought a look of love to her face. Eventually, the Alzheimer's Disease got worse and Joan died. During the time leading up to her death, Henry prayed every day, like he always did. Even when Joan was at her worse, he would always say, "God never forgets who Joan is."

Questions for Reflection

1. What memories do you have that form the
    foundation of your personality?

    _____

    _____

    _____

    _____

    _____

2. What have you done or seen someone do that
    has brought comfort to an Alzheimer's patient?

    _____

    _____

    _____

    _____

    _____

3. When caring for an Alzheimer's patient, especially
    in the later stages of the disease, how do you
    maintain their dignity?

    _____

    _____

    _____

    _____

    _____

Prayer for an Alzheimer's Patient

I am caring for a patient with Alzheimer's today
I give thanks for the memories
*   that are present today;*

*   For the moments when we can relate*
*   person to person.*

Help me to have patience during those times
*   when the illness prevents us from connecting.*

Help me to remember that You are present
*   in all things and in all experiences.*

Help me to remember that all the moments
*   I spend with this patient are precious.*

Prayer for an Orthopedic Patient

Remember the anatomy lessons in Nursing school?
Did you memorize the names of the bones in the
hands, or the muscles and their insertion points and
actions? I found all that stuff fascinating because I
was amazed at what the body can do. As a child,
I had all kinds of questions like:

How can a hand close into a fist?
What makes a knee bend?
How come you can't touch your right elbow with
your right hand?

After Nursing school, there were other questions like:

How do we fix this hand so that it closes again?
How do we get this knee to bend correctly?
How do we get this arm to straighten out right?

Usually, with the proper procedure and Nursing care,
the body will mend and normal activity will be
restored. And, once again, I am amazed at what the
body can do.

Questions for Reflection

It is easy to take bones for granted. In order to prevent this from happening, answer the following questions:

1. What are the tasks of daily living that would be different if your dominant hand was broken?

    _____
    _____
    _____
    _____

2. What would it be like to try to sleep right after a total hip replacement?

    _____
    _____
    _____
    _____

3. What would it be like to walk down the street with an arthritic knee?

    _____
    _____
    _____
    _____

Prayer for an Orthopedic Patient

*This patient is undergoing a procedure to fix his
(her) _____ (bone/joint).*

*Give health and strength to this area.
Allow the bone to mend,
the tendon to become strong,
and the joint to function normally.*

*Give patience to this patient to allow
the process of healing to occur*

and to prevent re-injury until full health returns.

your stories

chapter two

Discover Your Stories

We create ourselves out of the stories we tell about our lives, stories that impose purpose and meaning on experiences that often seem random and discontinuous.

Drew Gilpin Faust

How busy is your life? Many of us seem to spend our lives going from one event to another. In a typical day, we could start out running and not stop until we go to bed. Busyness seems to be the hallmark of our lives. It is as if the only reason we live is to go from activity to activity. When our life is this busy, we can forget the true purpose behind all this activity.

Nursing is also very busy. We can get so busy that we forget the reason why we do this work. Without remembering the deeper meaning behind our activities, Nursing becomes a series of tasks that become inconsequential. Drew Gilpin points out that when we don't remember the deeper meaning behind our activities, we become burnt out.

There are many ways that we can fight this sense of burnout. Adequate rest and nutrition, relaxation, mediation, and prayer are all effective. Creating and sharing a story is another way to connect with the deeper meaning of our lives. Stories that recall important moments can revitalize the way we work as nurses. Just the act of telling a story can enhance your outlook on Nursing. The following is a story told by a mental health nurse who attended one of our seminars. It exemplifies how a story can help you to connect with deeper meaning.

> *I was on the Open Unit when I heard the code alarm. (In mental health, a "code" is a physical restraint of a patient.) As I ran into the quiet room, I saw that a six-foot tall patient had meticulously removed the screws that held the cover over the room's radiator. He had ripped the radiator from the floor and was holding it over his head, about to throw it at the other nurse in the room.*

> *I had known the patient previously and had a joking relationship with him. I stepped into the room, cleared my throat, and said in my best Oliver Hardy voice, "Well, Stanley, here's another fine mess you've gotten us into." The patient laughed and relaxed his shoulders. I stepped close to him and asked him to listen closely to my voice.*

I asked him to slowly lower the radiator to the floor, which he did. Then, I asked him to sit in the corner of the quiet room away from the radiator. I kept talking to him, keeping his attention on me. I would say things like, "Bill, now the other nurses are going to get the other quiet room ready so we can walk over there." When the other room was ready, we walked over to the open QR with an escort of staff. He took some medication and fell asleep. I went back to the Open Unit and completed charting.

– Leslie Garfield, RN

As you read through this story, what words would you use to describe this nurse? When we ask that question in the seminar, we get answers like "competent", "cool-headed", and "decisive". The nurse, however, thought of herself as rather flighty and introverted. As the seminar discussed the story, her areas of competence became clearer to her. At one point in the discussion, she said, "I'm more competent than I thought I was." This story caused her to look at herself in a different way.

Remembering, crafting, and telling stories create meaning for people. Stories add focus to the randomness of life. In the words of sociologist Erving Goffman, stories become a "primary frame of reference." Goffman says that life is so complex that it must be looked at through a frame, much like a picture frame, which helps create a definition of life. This frame of reference can be used to interpret experiences, decide upon feelings, and direct our actions.

We use stories to help us make sense of the world. When we encounter some new experience, we search our memory for a story that is similar to help us understand the new experience. This process can happen so fast it can occur unconsciously. Remembering, crafting, and telling a story bring this unconscious process to the surface where the story can be fully understood. There are basically 4 types of stories: (See Chart 1)

	Empowering	Disempowering
Conscious	1	2
Unconscious	3	4

Chart 1

As you can see from Chart 1, stories can be unconscious or conscious, empowering or disempowering.

Quadrant 4 stories - *Disempowering Unconscious Stories* are those nagging voices and experiences that tear at our self esteem and abilities. Oftentimes, these stories are based on mistaken beliefs and opinions. These stories have powerful effects on behavior. Since they are unconscious, we are not able to change these behaviors without bringing the stories to the conscious level.

Quadrant 3 stories - *Empowering Unconscious Stories* are those stories that are secret sources of strength. These stories are helpful, but are unpredictable in their effect because they are in our unconscious mind.

Quadrant 2 stories - *Disempowering Conscious Stories* can actually be healthy in the long run. When a story is in the conscious mind, it can be examined for accuracy. This type of story can motivate people to make positive changes to their lives.

Quadrant 1 stories - *Empowering Conscious Stories* are stories we can use to help us deal with tough situations. They give us confidence and the ability to take on new challenges.

In this chapter, we outline a process you can use to create several different Quadrant 1 and 2 stories. Here is an example of this process at work. Several years ago, the following situation happened in one of our seminars. Participants were asked this question: "In your job, what is something that you would like to improve upon?" Participants then broke up into groups of two where this exchange occurred.

Participant 1: *I wish I could be more assertive. I get tired of being bullied by anyone and everyone. I have tried to learn to be assertive, but nothing has worked.*

Participant 2: *Why are you that way?*

Participant 1: *I don't know. I was always that way. My mother was always that way.*

Participant 2: *I wish we had more teamwork...*

The first participant was acting in a way she did not like. She was not being assertive and was unable to change her behavior. She only gave a brief indication of what may be a cause. After the session, she came up and told us that she remembered a story about her mother saying, "Good girls are quiet girls." This unconscious story created a frame of reference that disempowered her from being assertive. It was a Quadrant 4 story. When she started to tell the story, it became a Quadrant 2 where she became more aware of how it affected her behavior.

We then asked her to complete the exercise at the end of this chapter. When she had finished this exercise, she felt as if she had 5 other Quadrant 1 stories that showed her that she did not have to believe that "Good girls are quiet girls." She said, "I can become more assertive if I want."

We should give a few disclaimers at this point. This process is not therapy. When you remember craft, and tell a story about yourself, you highlight strengths and weaknesses that you already possess. Therapy deals with deeper issues that require the guidance of a skilled professional. While these two processes touch on similar issues, they are separate.

What follows is an exercise to help you discover your stories. In these exercises, you will try to remember stories about experiences that made you feel proud to be a nurse, demonstrated your knowledge, highlighted an accomplishment you achieved, demonstrated your compassion, or showed where you made a difference.

After you write a few lines describing these stories, use the accompanying chart to learn a little more from the story.

Once you have them written down, tell them to someone. After you do this several times, the stories become frames of reference for future events. The nurses who have completed this exercise have told us that they recall the stories when they need a sense of renewal and hope.

Discover Your Own Stories

Write a story about an experience that happened to you as a nurse which made you proud to be a nurse. (Use another page if necessary.)

_____

_____

_____

_____

_____

_____

_____

_____

_____

_____

_____

_____

_____

_____

_____

_____

_____

_____

_____

_____

_____

This grid is for the story that _____	List the obstacles you had to overcome:	What did you do to overcome these obstacles?	What happened as result of what you did?	What did you learn?

Write a story about an experience that happened to you as a nurse that demonstrated your knowledge.

_____
_____
_____
_____
_____
_____
_____
_____
_____
_____
_____
_____
_____
_____
_____
_____
_____
_____
_____
_____
_____
_____
_____
_____

Write a story about an experience that happened to
you as a nurse in which you accomplished something
few other people could have accomplished.

_____

_____

_____

_____

_____

_____

_____

_____

_____

_____

_____

_____

_____

_____

_____

_____

_____

_____

_____

_____

_____

_____

_____

Write a story about an experience that happened to you as a nurse that showed your compassion.

_____

_____

_____

_____

_____

_____

_____

_____

_____

Write a story about an experience or story that happened to you as a nurse in which you were effective at your job.

_____

_____

_____

_____

_____

_____

_____

_____

_____

_____

This grid is for the story that _____	List the obstacles you had to overcome:	What did you do to overcome these obstacles?	What happened as result of what you did?	What did you learn about yourself?

This grid is for the story that _____	List the obstacles you had to overcome:	What did you do to overcome these obstacles?	What happened as result of what you did?	What did you learn about yourself?

This grid is for the story that _____	List the obstacles you had to overcome:	What did you do to overcome these obstacles?	What happened as result of what you did?	What did you learn about yourself?

This grid is for the story that _____	List the obstacles you had to overcome:	What did you do to overcome these obstacles?	What happened as result of what you did?	What did you learn about yourself?

reflections

chapter three

Reflections on the Hands of a Nurse

The idea for this book came out a series of seminars called "Nursing Retreat Days". Nursing Retreat Day was carried out in partnership with Solution Seminars. During this retreat, the participants would tell stories about this profession called Nursing.

I began writing a series of reflections to capture the sentiment of these stories. As a presenter, I never seemed to lack the ability to use a lot of words. However, the reflections seemed to have tremendous meaning with very few words. There is an accompanying poster for each reflection. In this section, we will provide you the words for each reflection and sample of the accompanying poster. The posters may be purchased and a percentage of the sales will go to the support of Nursing education and other programs related to the improvement of healthcare. Please see the back of this book for ordering details.

The reflections that represent the specialty Nursing organizations rely heavily on feedback I have received from members of the national organizations that represent each of these specialties. When I tried to write a reflection that embodied these specialties without this feedback, I found my words were inadequate and superficial. Therefore, when I was unable to get feedback, I chose not to write a reflection. In subsequent editions, I hope to insert new entries that will represent these specialties.

As with any work, the feedback I received was only advisory in nature. Any offense or objections to the following reflections are my responsibility and not those of the organizations or nurses who provided feedback. I am grateful to all the nurses who offered assistance with this part of the book. Each conversation about this section reminded me that Nursing is truly a great profession full of wonderful people.

This reflection has received the most positive feedback, and we continue to get requests for the poster. In my opinion, it does the best job of capturing the sacredness of the profession called "Nursing."

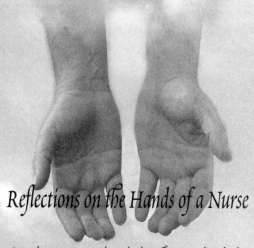

Reflections on the Hands of a Nurse

Let us take a moment to remember our hands. For these are no ordinary hands.
These are the hands of a nurse. These are the hands that feel the first breath
of a new born child. These are the hands that feel the last breath of a dying one.

These are the hands that bind the wounds that contain odor and pus.
These are the hands that insert tubes that bring healing to the body. These are the hands
that touch a forehead and tell, within a degree, normal or febrile. These are the hands
that feel a pulse and know fast or slow, weak or strong, effective or for naught.

These are the hands that clean unspeakable places on another person's body but do so
with dignity and respect which allow that person to feel like a human being.

These are also the hands of different people not just black or white, brown or yellow but all.
These are not the hands of male or female but both.

Other hands may build buildings or write books. Some hands may even pull the trigger or plunge the knife
but these are the hands of life. These are the hands that take up the task passed down
from so long ago-to bring healing to the sick, comfort to the afflicted, hope to the hopeless.

But these are not the hands of timid maidens who look for direction outside themselves
These are also the hands that can be clenched because sometimes some thing has got to change.
These are the hands of a nurse.

These are the hands that have the privilege of being at the bedside. That have the honor
to care and receive the joy of making a difference. For these are the hands of a nurse.
The hands of a person that does a job that not everyone can do. These are the hands of a nurse.

These are my hands

© 2002 Mark Darby

(Actual Poster 11x17)

Reflections on the Hands of a Nurse

Let us take a moment to remember our hands.
For these are no ordinary hands.
These are the hands of a nurse.

These are the hands that feel the first breath
   of a new born child.
These are the hands that feel the last breath
   of a dying one.

These are the hands that bind the wounds
   that contain odor and pus.
These are the hands that insert tubes that
   bring healing to the body.

These are the hands that touch a forehead and tell,
   within a degree, normal or febrile.
These are the hands that feel a pulse and know
   fast or slow, weak or strong, effective
   or for naught.

These are the hands that clean unspeakable places
  on another person's body but do so with dignity
  and respect which allow that person to feel
  like a human being.

These are also the hands of different people
  not just black or white, brown or yellow but all.
These are not the hands of male or female but both.

Other hands may build buildings or write books.
Some hands may even pull the trigger or plunge
  the knife but these are the hands of life.

These are the hands that take up the task
  passed down from so long ago – to bring healing
  to the sick, comfort to the afflicted, hope to the
  hopeless.

But these are not the hands of timid maidens
  who look for direction outside themselves.

These are also the hands that can be clenched
  because sometimes some thing has got to change.

These are the hands of a nurse.
These are the hands that have the privilege
    of being at the bedside.
For these are the hands of a nurse. The hands of a
    person that does a job that not everyone can do.
These are the hands of a nurse.

These are my hands.

The Work

The Work is the second reflection we used during the "Nursing Retreat Days." This reflection reminds me how rewarding Nursing is as a career. One of my first Nursing instructors said, "You will get more out of Nursing than you put in if you listen to your patients." There is a great deal of wisdom in those words.

The Work tells that the job we do as nurses affects more than just our patients.

Unfortunately, we do not have a poster for this reflection.

The Work

Joseph Conrad said, "I don't like to work...but I like what is in the work - the chance to find yourself." We often think of work as something that we do outside of ourselves, as something we do to pay the bills. But, the work we do also works on us.

When you first thought about being a nurse, there was someone who helped you realize that the work was desirable. The person who encouraged you was encouraged by someone else, who was encouraged by another until we get so far back we run into people like Florence Nightingale or Clara Barton.

When we reflect on people like Florence and Clara, we can begin to think that Nursing was formed by the heroic actions of extraordinary people. But Nursing was shaped by ordinary people. Ordinary people who were doing the same extraordinary work we are doing. It was not that they brought brilliance to the work but that the work helped them to become brilliant.

Now, we rightly honor Florence because of the contributions she made. Within six months of her arrival at Scutari during the Crimean War, the death rate in army hospitals fell from 42.7% to 2.2%. But, we forget that she was stubborn and bull-headed. The work helped her overcome all that.

Nursing is not a great profession because of the extraordinary deeds of a few individuals. Rather, it is great because it is the summation of a thousand ordinary acts by thousands of individuals. Walt Whitman, who was a nurse in the Civil War, wrote a poem called *Vigil Strange, I Kept One Night*. In it, Walt takes time away from the multiple tasks he must do as a nurse to provide an act of dignity to a dying soldier. The decent burial may have been an ordinary act of compassion, but it was the most important act that could be done for that soldier. For one brief moment, Walt was an extraordinary hero.

For the last century and a half, there have been hundreds of thousands of nurses who do the Work. The work of Nursing. And the work makes them heroes. For example, in the beginning of World War II, 81 nurses were on the Philippine Islands when it was attacked by the Japanese on Dec. 8, 1941. 81 nurses witnessed bombings, the battle for Corrigador, and the daily struggle for life. Some escaped, but most spent 37 months in a Japanese prison camp. Not one of them died in that camp. Not One. They say it was the work that kept them alive. The work gave them purpose, hope, and strength. It was the work that turned these ordinary people into extraordinary individuals.

Similarly, nurses continued to serve in Korea, Vietnam, and the Gulf War, and continue to serve on new fronts. In Vietnam, 11, 000 women served – 90% of them were nurses. There are 8 names of women on the Vietnam War Memorial–the Wall–on the Mall in Washington DC. And today there are new battlefields–Emergency Departments in New York, High Schools in Colorado. In all these battlefields, nurses, both men and women, perform great tasks and small tasks. But they all do The Work. The same work we do.

You know, the lamp, has been the symbol of Nursing for 150 years. It has always seemed kind of hokey to me. An image of a tireless saint going from patient to patient, offering comfort, seemed so different than the reality I experienced. But, I am beginning to change my mind about this lamp. It is not so much a lamp outside, but a light that burns inside us. A light that gives us heat and passion for our job. A fire that burns away our failures and tests our skills, making us better. It is the lamp inside that makes a nurse - a good nurse anyway.

The Door

Emergency Nursing has always been fascinating to me. As a psychiatric nurse, the ED seemed worlds away from my experience. I have often thought of the door to the ED as the symbol of this specialty. When you work in the ED, you never know what will come through the door, but you do have to be prepared for whatever it is.

When I contacted the Emergency Nurses Association about this project, I received tremendous help from several people. I want to thank Donna Massey, RN, MSN, CCNS, Chair of the ENA's Certification Board, as well as the numerous chairs of the state ENA chapters for their feedback. Several members of the ENA staff were a tremendous help, but Dale Gibbons deserves my special thanks.

If you would like to join the ENA, contact them at:
Emergency Nurses Association
915 Lee Street
Des Plaines, IL 60016
800-900-9659
or on the web at wwww.ena.org

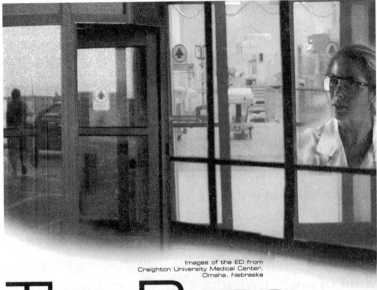

Images of the ED from
Creighton University Medical Center,
Omaha, Nebraska

The Door

Words for those who work in the ED

There is a door where I work – A door to the outside.

You never know who will come through the door; but when someone does, I help them. That is what I do.

Quickly, I assess and treat, listen and respond, and when I have done all I can do, I watch and wait and hope.

Sometimes a challenge comes through the door and I learn something new.

Sometimes, funny things come through that door, and I feel lighter.

Sometimes tragedy comes through the door, and I feel sad.

And sometimes, a miracle comes through the door, and I feel awe.

There are days when I feel I can handle anything that comes through the door.

And there are days when I want to quit. The paperwork and the bureaucracy get to me. On these days I seek out others who work with me and share some tears and some laughter. Then I feel better.

And I go back to work and answer the door.

© Mark Darby

www.mdarby.com • 402-451-3459

(Actual Poster 11x17)

The Door

Words for those who work in the ED

There is a door where I work – A door to the outside.

You never know who will come through the door;
   but when someone does, I help them.
   That is what I do.

Quickly, I assess and treat, listen and respond, and
   when I have done all I can do, I watch and wait
   and hope.

Sometimes a challenge comes through the door,
   and I learn something new.

Sometimes, funny things come through that door,
   and I feel lighter.

Sometimes tragedy comes through the door,
   and I feel sad.

And sometimes, a miracle comes through the door,
   and I feel awe.

There are days when I feel I can handle anything
   that comes through the door.

And there are days when I want to quit.
The paperwork and the bureaucracy get to me.
On these days I seek out others who work with
me and share some tears and some laughter. Then
I feel better.

And I go back to work and answer the door.

A Reflection on Medical Surgical Nursing

Medical Surgical nurses do almost any type of Nursing. The Med-Surg floor has become a place where almost any type of patient, with any level of acuity, can be found. This presents great challenges to nurses who work in this area. When I began to work on this reflection, the one characteristic of these nurses that seemed to stand out was the pride they felt for their jobs.

I received invaluable assistance in this reflection from Marlene Roman, RN, MSN, who is past president of the Academy of Medical Surgical Nurses. AMSN has a program called "Nurses Nurturing Nurses." This is the only specialty that has had two reflections written for them.

If you would like to find out more about the Academy of Medical Surgical Nurses, you may contact them at:

AMSN National Office
East Holly Avenue, PO Box 56
Pitman, NJ 08071-0056
856-256-2323 or
www.medsurgenurse.org

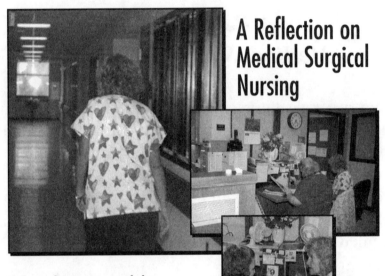

A Reflection on Medical Surgical Nursing

I never have a typical day...

It is not unusual for me to go to one room
and do wound care...
   and then a room with telemetry...
      then go to the next for a detox patient...
         followed by an out-of-control diabetic.

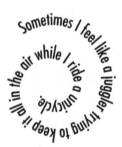

Sometimes I feel like a juggler trying to keep it all in the air while I ride a unicycle.

...But you know, I hardly ever drop anything,
that is because I am good at what I do.

Sometimes it seems that the better I get,
the more I am taken for granted.

I am expected to fill a depth of paperwork
and still give good care.

Someday this will all change. I know I may have to
give up something to enable these changes.

But one thing I will not give up...
I will not give up being a good nurse.

(Actual Poster 11x17)

A Reflection on Medical Surgical Nursing

I never have a typical day...
It is not unusual for me to go to one room
   and do wound care...
   and then a room with telemetry...
   then go to the next for a detox patient...
   followed by an out-of-control diabetic.

Sometimes I feel like a juggler trying to
   keep it all in the air while I ride a unicycle.

...But you know, I hardly ever drop anything,
that is because I am good at what I do.

Sometimes it seems that the better I get,
   the more I am taken for granted.
I am expected to fill a depth of paperwork and
   still give good care.

Someday this will all change. I know I may have
   to give up something to enable these changes.

But one thing I will not give up...
I will not give up being a good nurse.

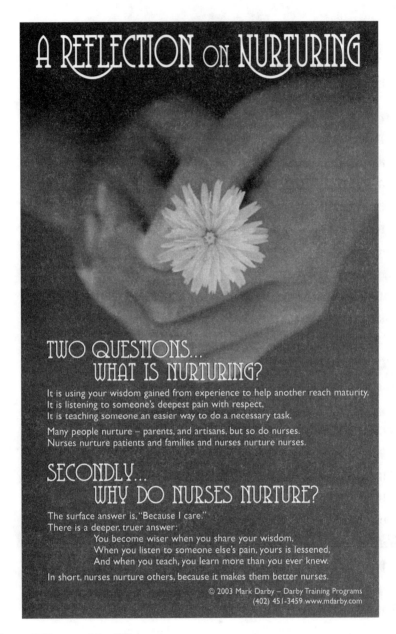

(Actual Poster 11x17)

A Reflection on Nurturing

Two Questions...
What is Nurturing?

It is using your wisdom gained from experience
   to help another reach maturity,
It is listening to someone's deepest pain with respect,
It is teaching someone an easier way
   to do a necessary task.

Many people nurture - parents, and artisans,
   but so do nurses.
Nurses nurture patients and families and
   nurses nurture nurses.

Secondly, Why do Nurses Nurture?

The surface answer is, "Because I care."
There is a deeper, truer answer:
You become wiser when you share your wisdom,
When you listen to someone else's pain,
   yours is lessened,

And when you teach, you learn more
   than you ever knew.

In short, nurses nurture others,
   because it makes them better nurses.

The Blur

School Nursing is a joy. The ability to help children be ready to learn is admirable and life-giving. The rewards for this work are great, but the challenges are many. The pay is amongst the lowest wages in Nursing and the ratio of school nurse to students continues to increase.

Still, school nurses continue to thrive and to have a positive effect upon children. The professional organization representing school nurses can be reached at:

National Association of School Nurses
PO Box 1300
Scarborough, ME 04070
877-627-6476
www.nasn.org

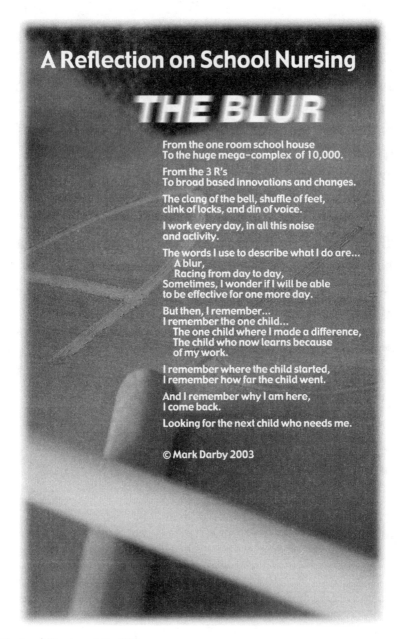

(Actual Poster 11x17)

The Blur

From the one room school house
  To the huge mega-complex of 10,000.
From the 3 R's
  To broad based innovations and changes.
The clang of the bell, shuffle of feet,
  clink of locks, and din of voice.

I work every day, in all this noise and activity.

The words I use to describe what I do are...
A blur,
Racing from day to day,
Sometimes, I wonder if I will be able to be effective
  for one more day.

But then,
  I remember...
  I remember the one child...

The one child where I made a difference,
The child who now learns because of my work.

I remember where the child started,
I remember how far the child went.
   And I remember why I am here,
   I come back.
   Looking for the next child who needs me.

A Reflection on GI Nursing

When I started this reflection, I asked several GI nurses to tell me about GI Nursing. I received page after page of GI humor. They were some of the most humorous stories I remember. The theme of humor formed the basis for this reflection.

If you would like to contact the Society for Gastroenterology Nurses and Associates, you can reach them at:

SGNA
401 North Michigan Ave.
Chicago, IL 60611-4267
800-245-7462
www.sgna.org

A Reflection on GI Nursing

Jokes and Puns, Guffaws and Giggles.
And disgusted looks on faces.

I get them all and I get them in the strangest places...
        At church
        At a party
        In a store

And I get them from all kinds of people...
        Men and women
        White and blue collar
        Young and old

  I get it all the time — except from patients

It seems that jokes stop when you sit on the table
and we examine you.

I guess no one takes the GI tract seriously
until it stops working

Yet when you sit there exposing areas
that make you vulnerable...
        I crack a joke
        I also smile, and encourage,
        I'm business-like and make it all painless as possible

And when you're done, you look at me without
        A joke
        A guffaw
        Or a disgusted look

          And you say thanks

          Mark Darby, RN

(Actual Poster 11x17)

A Reflection on
GI Nursing

Jokes and Puns, Guffaws and Giggles.
 And disgusted looks on faces.

I get them all and I get them in the strangest places...
 At church
 At a party
 In a store

And I get them from all kinds of people...
 Men and women
 White and blue collar
 Young and old

I get it all the time – except from patients

It seems that jokes stop when you
 sit on the table and we examine you.

I guess no one takes the GI tract seriously
 until it stops working

Yet when you sit there exposing areas
    that make you vulnerable... I crack a joke

I also smile, and encourage, and calm
I'm business-like and make it all
    as painless as possible

And when you're done, you look at me without
    A joke
    A guffaw
    Or a disgusted look

And you say thanks

The Covenant

Working with the elderly is a special undertaking.
This group of patients has done much with their
lives. In many ways, this type of Nursing is sacred.
Yet, reimbursement, staffing ratios, and regulations
make this work difficult and prone to burnout. This
reflection was designed to help those who work with
the elderly remember why they do what they do.
Hopefully by remembering, they will become
refreshed and strengthened.

Unlike the other reflections, this was not written in
consultation with a specialty Nursing organization.
It was written with the advice of several nurses who
work in long-term care organizations. I am grateful
for their help.

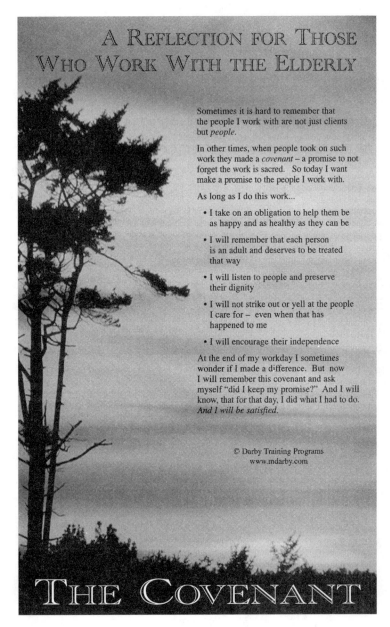

(Actual Poster 11x17)

145

The Covenant
(A Reflection for Those Who Work With the Elderly)

Sometimes it is hard to remember that the
  people I work with are not just clients
  but *people*.

In other times, when people took on such work
  they made a *covenant* - a promise
  to not forget the work is sacred.

So today I want make a promise to the people
  I work with.

As long as I do this work...
  I take on an obligation to help them
  be as happy and as healthy as they can be

  I will remember that each person is an adult
  and deserves to be treated that way

  I will listen to people and preserve their dignity

  I will not strike out or yell at the people
  I care for - even when that has happened to me

I will encourage their independence

At the end of my workday I sometimes wonder
   if I made a difference. But now I will remember
   this covenant and ask myself, "Did I keep my
   promise?"

And I will know, that for that day, I did what
   I had to do

And I will be satisfied.

A Reflection on
Occupational Health Nursing

Occupational Health Nursing is very foreign to me.
I hurt my back once and went to the employee
health nurse for an exam. This brief encounter did
not give me a true understanding of the complexity
of this specialty.

That is why I am grateful for the assistance of Marcia
Noble of the American Association of Occupational
Health Nursing. If you would like to join AAOHN, you
can contact them at:

AAOHN
2920 Brandywine Rd. Suite 100
Atlanta, GA 30341
(770) 455-7757
www.aaohn.org

A Reflection on
Occupational Health Nursing

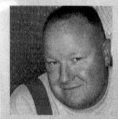

They tell me...
I'm a carpenter or
I'm a steamfitter or
I'm a mailman or
I'm a packing house worker or
I'm a teacher or
Any number of other occupations.
And I always reply *"I'm a nurse."*
They work day in and day out
To make things
To provide services
To haul cargo

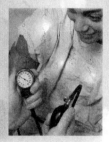

They do many things.
I look at how things are done to make them more effective,
to make them safe, to make their job more efficient
I educate and advocate for their health. I talk to them about
doing things differently, so they can go home alive and well
Sometimes I have to bandage them, and care for their injuries.
Other times I help them get the most efficient and effective
care. I help them navigate successfully through the maze of
health care.
I do all this under budget and on time
I do all these things because the last thing I want them to say is...
Because of my injuries, I can't work
This is what I do

But every time they say something like...
I'm a cook or
I'm an electrician or
I'm a steelworker,
They can say that is because
I'm a nurse and I do my job.

© 2003 Mark Darby

(Actual Poster 11x17)

A Reflection on Occupational Health Nursing

They tell me...
  I'm a carpenter or
  I'm a steamfitter or
  I'm a mailman or
  I'm a packing house worker or
  I'm a teacher or
  Any number of other occupations.

And I always reply, "I'm a nurse."

They work day in and day out
  To make things
  To provide services
  To haul cargo
They do many things.

I look at how things are done to make them more effective, to make them safe, to make their job more efficient

I educate and advocate for their health. I talk to them about doing things differently, so they can go home alive and well

Sometimes I have to bandage them, and care for
their injuries. Other times I help them get the most
efficient and effective care. I help them navigate
successfully through the maze of health care.

I do all this under budget and on time
I do all these things because the last thing I want
them to say is...
    Because of my injuries, I can't work
This is what I do.

But every time they say something like...
    I'm a cook or
    I'm an electrician or
    I'm a steelworker,

They can say that because I'm a nurse
    and I do my job.

A Reflection on Psychiatric Nursing

This and the next reflection are based largely on my own experiences. I never wanted to do any other type of Nursing except Mental Health Nursing. When I tell people I am a psych nurse, they say, "I could never do psych." In my opinion, it is the best type of Nursing.

I like it because your own skill and empathy are the most important tools, and there are no machines that beep. When machines beep, I think I am going to break something.

I am much more comfortable with a live human being. When I have shared this reflection with other psych nurses, they have enjoyed it. I hope you enjoy it as well.

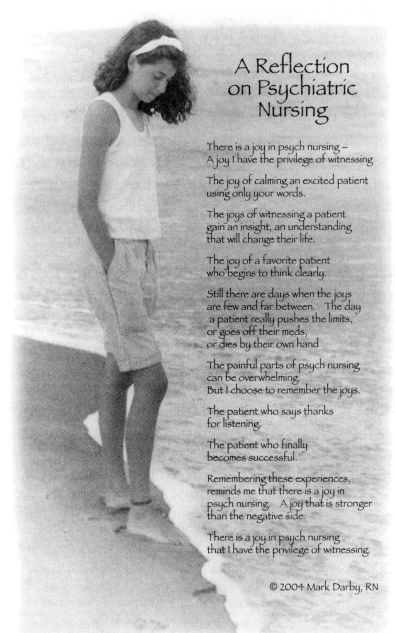

A Reflection
on Psychiatric
Nursing

There is a joy in psych nursing –
A joy I have the privilege of witnessing

The joy of calming an excited patient
using only your words.

The joys of witnessing a patient
gain an insight, an understanding
that will change their life.

The joy of a favorite patient
who begins to think clearly.

Still there are days when the joys
are few and far between.   The day
a patient really pushes the limits,
or goes off their meds,
or dies by their own hand

The painful parts of psych nursing
can be overwhelming.
But I choose to remember the joys.

The patient who says thanks
for listening.

The patient who finally
becomes successful.

Remembering these experiences,
reminds me that there is a joy in
psych nursing.   A joy that is stronger
than the negative side.

There is a joy in psych nursing
that I have the privilege of witnessing.

© 2004 Mark Darby, RN

(Actual Poster 11x17)

A Reflection on Psychiatric Nursing

There is a joy in psych nursing –
 A joy I have the privilege of witnessing

  The joy of calming an excited patient
  using only your words.

  The joys of witnessing a patient gain an insight,
  an understanding that will change their life

The joy of a favorite patient who begins
 to think clearly.

Still there are days when the joys are
 few and far between.

The day a patient really pushes the limits,
 or goes off their meds, or
 dies by their own hand

The painful parts of psych nursing can be overwhelming.
 But, I choose to remember the joys.

The patient who says thanks for listening.
The patient who finally becomes successful.

Remembering these experiences,
   reminds me that there is a joy in psych nursing.

A joy that is stronger than the negative side.

There is a joy in psych nursing
   that I have the privilege of witnessing.

A Reflection on
Home Health Nursing

On a whim, I took a part time job with the Visiting Nurses Association in the early 90's. I loved it. It is a special type of Nursing. The industry has undergone great changes in the last decade, but the essential work, the work of Nursing, is special.

It felt like an adventure. You meet all kinds of people – both pleasant and challenging – when you do that job. The autonomy and the ability to interact on a one-on-one basis is special. I treasure the time I spent in this specialty.

A Reflection on Home Health Nursing

It is different to do nursing in someone's home. In a home you are not in control - you don't have the advantage. In a home you are a guest.

This status creates an intimate atmosphere where you get to know your client not just as a patient but as a human being.

You are in the place where the precious memories and experiences are stored.

And in restoring health in the home, you become part of those memories.

When I think of home health in this way, I become more respectful of my responsibility, more mindful of the obligation I bear.

And I remember the honor I enjoy - the honor of giving care and restoring health in someone's home.

© Mark Darby, RN

(Actual Poster 11x17)

A Reflection on Home Health Nursing

It is different to do nursing in someone's home.
In a home you are not in control – you don't have
  the advantage.

In a home you are a guest.

This status creates an intimate atmosphere
  where you get to know your client
    not just as a patient but also as a human being.

You are in the place where the precious memories
  and experiences are stored.

And in restoring health in the home,
  you become part of those memories.

When I think of home health in this way,
  I become more respectful of my responsibility,
  more mindful of the obligation I bear.

And I remember the honor I enjoy –
  the honor of giving care and restoring health
  in someone's home.